This book belongs

Name: _____

Telephone: _____

Address: _____
_____

In case of emergency please contact:

Name: _____

Telephone: _____

Address: _____
_____

Week of

	Breakfast		Lunch		Dinner		Night
	before	after	before	after	before	after	before
MONDAY							

Notes:

	Breakfast		Lunch		Dinner		Night
	before	after	before	after	before	after	before
TUESDAY							

Notes:

	Breakfast		Lunch		Dinner		Night
	before	after	before	after	before	after	before
WEDNESDAY							

Notes:

	Breakfast		Lunch		Dinner		Night
	before	after	before	after	before	after	before
THURSDAY							

Notes:

	Breakfast		Lunch		Dinner		Night
	before	after	before	after	before	after	before
FRIDAY							

Notes:

	Breakfast		Lunch		Dinner		Night
	before	after	before	after	before	after	before
SATURDAY							

Notes:

	Breakfast		Lunch		Dinner		Night
	before	after	before	after	before	after	before
SUNDAY							

Notes:

Week of

	Breakfast		Lunch		Dinner		Night
	before	after	before	after	before	after	before
MONDAY							

Notes:

	before	after	before	after	before	after	before
TUESDAY							

Notes:

	before	after	before	after	before	after	before
WEDNESDAY							

Notes:

	before	after	before	after	before	after	before
THURSDAY							

Notes:

	before	after	before	after	before	after	before
FRIDAY							

Notes:

	before	after	before	after	before	after	before
SATURDAY							

Notes:

	before	after	before	after	before	after	before
SUNDAY							

Notes:

Week of

	Breakfast		Lunch		Dinner		Night
	before	after	before	after	before	after	before
MONDAY							

Notes:

	before	after	before	after	before	after	before
TUESDAY							

Notes:

	before	after	before	after	before	after	before
WEDNESDAY							

Notes:

	before	after	before	after	before	after	before
THURSDAY							

Notes:

	before	after	before	after	before	after	before
FRIDAY							

Notes:

	before	after	before	after	before	after	before
SATURDAY							

Notes:

	before	after	before	after	before	after	before
SUNDAY							

Notes:

Week of

	Breakfast		Lunch		Dinner		Night
MONDAY	before	after	before	after	before	after	before

Notes:

TUESDAY	before	after	before	after	before	after	before

Notes:

WEDNESDAY	before	after	before	after	before	after	before

Notes:

THURSDAY	before	after	before	after	before	after	before

Notes:

FRIDAY	before	after	before	after	before	after	before

Notes:

SATURDAY	before	after	before	after	before	after	before

Notes:

SUNDAY	before	after	before	after	before	after	before

Notes:

Week of

	Breakfast		Lunch		Dinner		Night
	before	after	before	after	before	after	before
MONDAY							

Notes:

	before	after	before	after	before	after	before
TUESDAY							

Notes:

	before	after	before	after	before	after	before
WEDNESDAY							

Notes:

	before	after	before	after	before	after	before
THURSDAY							

Notes:

	before	after	before	after	before	after	before
FRIDAY							

Notes:

	before	after	before	after	before	after	before
SATURDAY							

Notes:

	before	after	before	after	before	after	before
SUNDAY							

Notes:

Week of

	Breakfast		Lunch		Dinner		Night
	before	after	before	after	before	after	before
MONDAY							

Notes:

	before	after	before	after	before	after	before
TUESDAY							

Notes:

	before	after	before	after	before	after	before
WEDNESDAY							

Notes:

	before	after	before	after	before	after	before
THURSDAY							

Notes:

	before	after	before	after	before	after	before
FRIDAY							

Notes:

	before	after	before	after	before	after	before
SATURDAY							

Notes:

	before	after	before	after	before	after	before
SUNDAY							

Notes:

Week of

	Breakfast		Lunch		Dinner		Night
	before	after	before	after	before	after	before
MONDAY							

Notes:

	before	after	before	after	before	after	before
TUESDAY							

Notes:

	before	after	before	after	before	after	before
WEDNESDAY							

Notes:

	before	after	before	after	before	after	before
THURSDAY							

Notes:

	before	after	before	after	before	after	before
FRIDAY							

Notes:

	before	after	before	after	before	after	before
SATURDAY							

Notes:

	before	after	before	after	before	after	before
SUNDAY							

Notes:

Week of

	Breakfast		Lunch		Dinner		Night
	before	after	before	after	before	after	before
MONDAY							
Notes:							
TUESDAY	before	after	before	after	before	after	before
Notes:							
WEDNESDAY	before	after	before	after	before	after	before
Notes:							
THURSDAY	before	after	before	after	before	after	before
Notes:							
FRIDAY	before	after	before	after	before	after	before
Notes:							
SATURDAY	before	after	before	after	before	after	before
Notes:							
SUNDAY	before	after	before	after	before	after	before
Notes:							

Week of

	Breakfast		Lunch		Dinner		Night
	before	after	before	after	before	after	before
MONDAY							

Notes:

	before	after	before	after	before	after	before
TUESDAY							

Notes:

	before	after	before	after	before	after	before
WEDNESDAY							

Notes:

	before	after	before	after	before	after	before
THURSDAY							

Notes:

	before	after	before	after	before	after	before
FRIDAY							

Notes:

	before	after	before	after	before	after	before
SATURDAY							

Notes:

	before	after	before	after	before	after	before
SUNDAY							

Notes:

Week of

	Breakfast		Lunch		Dinner		Night
	before	after	before	after	before	after	before
MONDAY							

Notes:

	before	after	before	after	before	after	before
TUESDAY							

Notes:

	before	after	before	after	before	after	before
WEDNESDAY							

Notes:

	before	after	before	after	before	after	before
THURSDAY							

Notes:

	before	after	before	after	before	after	before
FRIDAY							

Notes:

	before	after	before	after	before	after	before
SATURDAY							

Notes:

	before	after	before	after	before	after	before
SUNDAY							

Notes:

Week of

	Breakfast		Lunch		Dinner		Night
	before	after	before	after	before	after	before
MONDAY							

Notes:

	before	after	before	after	before	after	before
TUESDAY							

Notes:

	before	after	before	after	before	after	before
WEDNESDAY							

Notes:

	before	after	before	after	before	after	before
THURSDAY							

Notes:

	before	after	before	after	before	after	before
FRIDAY							

Notes:

	before	after	before	after	before	after	before
SATURDAY							

Notes:

	before	after	before	after	before	after	before
SUNDAY							

Notes:

Week of

	Breakfast		Lunch		Dinner		Night
	before	after	before	after	before	after	before
MONDAY							
Notes:							
TUESDAY	before	after	before	after	before	after	before
Notes:							
WEDNESDAY	before	after	before	after	before	after	before
Notes:							
THURSDAY	before	after	before	after	before	after	before
Notes:							
FRIDAY	before	after	before	after	before	after	before
Notes:							
SATURDAY	before	after	before	after	before	after	before
Notes:							
SUNDAY	before	after	before	after	before	after	before
Notes:							

Week of

	Breakfast		Lunch		Dinner		Night
	before	after	before	after	before	after	before
MONDAY							

Notes:

	before	after	before	after	before	after	before
TUESDAY							

Notes:

	before	after	before	after	before	after	before
WEDNESDAY							

Notes:

	before	after	before	after	before	after	before
THURSDAY							

Notes:

	before	after	before	after	before	after	before
FRIDAY							

Notes:

	before	after	before	after	before	after	before
SATURDAY							

Notes:

	before	after	before	after	before	after	before
SUNDAY							

Notes:

Week of

	Breakfast		Lunch		Dinner		Night
MONDAY	before	after	before	after	before	after	before
Notes:							
TUESDAY	before	after	before	after	before	after	before
Notes:							
WEDNESDAY	before	after	before	after	before	after	before
Notes:							
THURSDAY	before	after	before	after	before	after	before
Notes:							
FRIDAY	before	after	before	after	before	after	before
Notes:							
SATURDAY	before	after	before	after	before	after	before
Notes:							
SUNDAY	before	after	before	after	before	after	before
Notes:							

Week of

	Breakfast		Lunch		Dinner		Night
	before	after	before	after	before	after	before
MONDAY							

Notes:

	before	after	before	after	before	after	before
TUESDAY							

Notes:

	before	after	before	after	before	after	before
WEDNESDAY							

Notes:

	before	after	before	after	before	after	before
THURSDAY							

Notes:

	before	after	before	after	before	after	before
FRIDAY							

Notes:

	before	after	before	after	before	after	before
SATURDAY							

Notes:

	before	after	before	after	before	after	before
SUNDAY							

Notes:

Week of

	Breakfast		Lunch		Dinner		Night
	before	after	before	after	before	after	before
MONDAY							

Notes:

	before	after	before	after	before	after	before
TUESDAY							

Notes:

	before	after	before	after	before	after	before
WEDNESDAY							

Notes:

	before	after	before	after	before	after	before
THURSDAY							

Notes:

	before	after	before	after	before	after	before
FRIDAY							

Notes:

	before	after	before	after	before	after	before
SATURDAY							

Notes:

	before	after	before	after	before	after	before
SUNDAY							

Notes:

Week of

	Breakfast		Lunch		Dinner		Night
	before	after	before	after	before	after	before
MONDAY							

Notes:

	before	after	before	after	before	after	before
TUESDAY							

Notes:

	before	after	before	after	before	after	before
WEDNESDAY							

Notes:

	before	after	before	after	before	after	before
THURSDAY							

Notes:

	before	after	before	after	before	after	before
FRIDAY							

Notes:

	before	after	before	after	before	after	before
SATURDAY							

Notes:

	before	after	before	after	before	after	before
SUNDAY							

Notes:

Week of

	Breakfast		Lunch		Dinner		Night
	before	after	before	after	before	after	before
MONDAY							
Notes:							
TUESDAY	before	after	before	after	before	after	before
Notes:							
WEDNESDAY	before	after	before	after	before	after	before
Notes:							
THURSDAY	before	after	before	after	before	after	before
Notes:							
FRIDAY	before	after	before	after	before	after	before
Notes:							
SATURDAY	before	after	before	after	before	after	before
Notes:							
SUNDAY	before	after	before	after	before	after	before
Notes:							

Week of

	Breakfast		Lunch		Dinner		Night
	before	after	before	after	before	after	before
MONDAY							

Notes:

	before	after	before	after	before	after	before
TUESDAY							

Notes:

	before	after	before	after	before	after	before
WEDNESDAY							

Notes:

	before	after	before	after	before	after	before
THURSDAY							

Notes:

	before	after	before	after	before	after	before
FRIDAY							

Notes:

	before	after	before	after	before	after	before
SATURDAY							

Notes:

	before	after	before	after	before	after	before
SUNDAY							

Notes:

Week of

	Breakfast		Lunch		Dinner		Night
	before	after	before	after	before	after	before
MONDAY							

Notes:

	before	after	before	after	before	after	before
TUESDAY							

Notes:

	before	after	before	after	before	after	before
WEDNESDAY							

Notes:

	before	after	before	after	before	after	before
THURSDAY							

Notes:

	before	after	before	after	before	after	before
FRIDAY							

Notes:

	before	after	before	after	before	after	before
SATURDAY							

Notes:

	before	after	before	after	before	after	before
SUNDAY							

Notes:

Week of

	Breakfast		Lunch		Dinner		Night
	before	after	before	after	before	after	before
MONDAY							
Notes:							
TUESDAY	before	after	before	after	before	after	before
Notes:							
WEDNESDAY	before	after	before	after	before	after	before
Notes:							
THURSDAY	before	after	before	after	before	after	before
Notes:							
FRIDAY	before	after	before	after	before	after	before
Notes:							
SATURDAY	before	after	before	after	before	after	before
Notes:							
SUNDAY	before	after	before	after	before	after	before
Notes:							

Week of

	Breakfast		Lunch		Dinner		Night
	before	after	before	after	before	after	before
MONDAY							

Notes:

	before	after	before	after	before	after	before
TUESDAY							

Notes:

	before	after	before	after	before	after	before
WEDNESDAY							

Notes:

	before	after	before	after	before	after	before
THURSDAY							

Notes:

	before	after	before	after	before	after	before
FRIDAY							

Notes:

	before	after	before	after	before	after	before
SATURDAY							

Notes:

	before	after	before	after	before	after	before
SUNDAY							

Notes:

Week of

	Breakfast		Lunch		Dinner		Night
	before	after	before	after	before	after	before
MONDAY							

Notes:

	before	after	before	after	before	after	before
TUESDAY							

Notes:

	before	after	before	after	before	after	before
WEDNESDAY							

Notes:

	before	after	before	after	before	after	before
THURSDAY							

Notes:

	before	after	before	after	before	after	before
FRIDAY							

Notes:

	before	after	before	after	before	after	before
SATURDAY							

Notes:

	before	after	before	after	before	after	before
SUNDAY							

Notes:

Week of

	Breakfast		Lunch		Dinner		Night
	before	after	before	after	before	after	before
MONDAY							

Notes:

	before	after	before	after	before	after	before
TUESDAY							

Notes:

	before	after	before	after	before	after	before
WEDNESDAY							

Notes:

	before	after	before	after	before	after	before
THURSDAY							

Notes:

	before	after	before	after	before	after	before
FRIDAY							

Notes:

	before	after	before	after	before	after	before
SATURDAY							

Notes:

	before	after	before	after	before	after	before
SUNDAY							

Notes:

Week of

	Breakfast		Lunch		Dinner		Night
	before	after	before	after	before	after	before
MONDAY							

Notes:

	before	after	before	after	before	after	before
TUESDAY							

Notes:

	before	after	before	after	before	after	before
WEDNESDAY							

Notes:

	before	after	before	after	before	after	before
THURSDAY							

Notes:

	before	after	before	after	before	after	before
FRIDAY							

Notes:

	before	after	before	after	before	after	before
SATURDAY							

Notes:

	before	after	before	after	before	after	before
SUNDAY							

Notes:

Week of

	Breakfast		Lunch		Dinner		Night
	before	after	before	after	before	after	before
MONDAY							

Notes:

	before	after	before	after	before	after	before
TUESDAY							

Notes:

	before	after	before	after	before	after	before
WEDNESDAY							

Notes:

	before	after	before	after	before	after	before
THURSDAY							

Notes:

	before	after	before	after	before	after	before
FRIDAY							

Notes:

	before	after	before	after	before	after	before
SATURDAY							

Notes:

	before	after	before	after	before	after	before
SUNDAY							

Notes:

Week of

	Breakfast		Lunch		Dinner		Night
	before	after	before	after	before	after	before
MONDAY							

Notes:

	before	after	before	after	before	after	before
TUESDAY							

Notes:

	before	after	before	after	before	after	before
WEDNESDAY							

Notes:

	before	after	before	after	before	after	before
THURSDAY							

Notes:

	before	after	before	after	before	after	before
FRIDAY							

Notes:

	before	after	before	after	before	after	before
SATURDAY							

Notes:

	before	after	before	after	before	after	before
SUNDAY							

Notes:

Week of

	Breakfast		Lunch		Dinner		Night
	before	after	before	after	before	after	before
MONDAY							
Notes:							
TUESDAY	before	after	before	after	before	after	before
Notes:							
WEDNESDAY	before	after	before	after	before	after	before
Notes:							
THURSDAY	before	after	before	after	before	after	before
Notes:							
FRIDAY	before	after	before	after	before	after	before
Notes:							
SATURDAY	before	after	before	after	before	after	before
Notes:							
SUNDAY	before	after	before	after	before	after	before
Notes:							

Week of

	Breakfast		Lunch		Dinner		Night
	before	after	before	after	before	after	before
MONDAY							
Notes:							
TUESDAY	before	after	before	after	before	after	before
Notes:							
WEDNESDAY	before	after	before	after	before	after	before
Notes:							
THURSDAY	before	after	before	after	before	after	before
Notes:							
FRIDAY	before	after	before	after	before	after	before
Notes:							
SATURDAY	before	after	before	after	before	after	before
Notes:							
SUNDAY	before	after	before	after	before	after	before
Notes:							

Week of

	Breakfast		Lunch		Dinner		Night
	before	after	before	after	before	after	before
MONDAY							

Notes:

	before	after	before	after	before	after	before
TUESDAY							

Notes:

	before	after	before	after	before	after	before
WEDNESDAY							

Notes:

	before	after	before	after	before	after	before
THURSDAY							

Notes:

	before	after	before	after	before	after	before
FRIDAY							

Notes:

	before	after	before	after	before	after	before
SATURDAY							

Notes:

	before	after	before	after	before	after	before
SUNDAY							

Notes:

Week of

	Breakfast		Lunch		Dinner		Night
MONDAY	before	after	before	after	before	after	before

Notes:

	Breakfast		Lunch		Dinner		Night
TUESDAY	before	after	before	after	before	after	before

Notes:

	Breakfast		Lunch		Dinner		Night
WEDNESDAY	before	after	before	after	before	after	before

Notes:

	Breakfast		Lunch		Dinner		Night
THURSDAY	before	after	before	after	before	after	before

Notes:

	Breakfast		Lunch		Dinner		Night
FRIDAY	before	after	before	after	before	after	before

Notes:

	Breakfast		Lunch		Dinner		Night
SATURDAY	before	after	before	after	before	after	before

Notes:

	Breakfast		Lunch		Dinner		Night
SUNDAY	before	after	before	after	before	after	before

Notes:

Week of

	Breakfast		Lunch		Dinner		Night
MONDAY	before	after	before	after	before	after	before

Notes:

TUESDAY	before	after	before	after	before	after	before

Notes:

WEDNESDAY	before	after	before	after	before	after	before

Notes:

THURSDAY	before	after	before	after	before	after	before

Notes:

FRIDAY	before	after	before	after	before	after	before

Notes:

SATURDAY	before	after	before	after	before	after	before

Notes:

SUNDAY	before	after	before	after	before	after	before

Notes:

Week of

	Breakfast		Lunch		Dinner		Night
	before	after	before	after	before	after	before
MONDAY							

Notes:

	before	after	before	after	before	after	before
TUESDAY							

Notes:

	before	after	before	after	before	after	before
WEDNESDAY							

Notes:

	before	after	before	after	before	after	before
THURSDAY							

Notes:

	before	after	before	after	before	after	before
FRIDAY							

Notes:

	before	after	before	after	before	after	before
SATURDAY							

Notes:

	before	after	before	after	before	after	before
SUNDAY							

Notes:

Week of

	Breakfast		Lunch		Dinner		Night
	before	after	before	after	before	after	before
MONDAY							

Notes:

	before	after	before	after	before	after	before
TUESDAY							

Notes:

	before	after	before	after	before	after	before
WEDNESDAY							

Notes:

	before	after	before	after	before	after	before
THURSDAY							

Notes:

	before	after	before	after	before	after	before
FRIDAY							

Notes:

	before	after	before	after	before	after	before
SATURDAY							

Notes:

	before	after	before	after	before	after	before
SUNDAY							

Notes:

Week of

	Breakfast		Lunch		Dinner		Night
	before	after	before	after	before	after	before
MONDAY							

Notes:

	before	after	before	after	before	after	before
TUESDAY							

Notes:

	before	after	before	after	before	after	before
WEDNESDAY							

Notes:

	before	after	before	after	before	after	before
THURSDAY							

Notes:

	before	after	before	after	before	after	before
FRIDAY							

Notes:

	before	after	before	after	before	after	before
SATURDAY							

Notes:

	before	after	before	after	before	after	before
SUNDAY							

Notes:

Week of

	Breakfast		Lunch		Dinner		Night
	before	after	before	after	before	after	before
MONDAY							

Notes:

	before	after	before	after	before	after	before
TUESDAY							

Notes:

	before	after	before	after	before	after	before
WEDNESDAY							

Notes:

	before	after	before	after	before	after	before
THURSDAY							

Notes:

	before	after	before	after	before	after	before
FRIDAY							

Notes:

	before	after	before	after	before	after	before
SATURDAY							

Notes:

	before	after	before	after	before	after	before
SUNDAY							

Notes:

Week of

	Breakfast		Lunch		Dinner		Night
	before	after	before	after	before	after	before
MONDAY							

Notes:

	before	after	before	after	before	after	before
TUESDAY							

Notes:

	before	after	before	after	before	after	before
WEDNESDAY							

Notes:

	before	after	before	after	before	after	before
THURSDAY							

Notes:

	before	after	before	after	before	after	before
FRIDAY							

Notes:

	before	after	before	after	before	after	before
SATURDAY							

Notes:

	before	after	before	after	before	after	before
SUNDAY							

Notes:

Week of

	Breakfast		Lunch		Dinner		Night
	before	after	before	after	before	after	before
MONDAY							

Notes:

	before	after	before	after	before	after	before
TUESDAY							

Notes:

	before	after	before	after	before	after	before
WEDNESDAY							

Notes:

	before	after	before	after	before	after	before
THURSDAY							

Notes:

	before	after	before	after	before	after	before
FRIDAY							

Notes:

	before	after	before	after	before	after	before
SATURDAY							

Notes:

	before	after	before	after	before	after	before
SUNDAY							

Notes:

Week of

	Breakfast		Lunch		Dinner		Night
	before	after	before	after	before	after	before
MONDAY							

Notes:

	before	after	before	after	before	after	before
TUESDAY							

Notes:

	before	after	before	after	before	after	before
WEDNESDAY							

Notes:

	before	after	before	after	before	after	before
THURSDAY							

Notes:

	before	after	before	after	before	after	before
FRIDAY							

Notes:

	before	after	before	after	before	after	before
SATURDAY							

Notes:

	before	after	before	after	before	after	before
SUNDAY							

Notes:

Week of

	Breakfast		Lunch		Dinner		Night
	before	after	before	after	before	after	before
MONDAY							

Notes:

	before	after	before	after	before	after	before
TUESDAY							

Notes:

	before	after	before	after	before	after	before
WEDNESDAY							

Notes:

	before	after	before	after	before	after	before
THURSDAY							

Notes:

	before	after	before	after	before	after	before
FRIDAY							

Notes:

	before	after	before	after	before	after	before
SATURDAY							

Notes:

	before	after	before	after	before	after	before
SUNDAY							

Notes:

Week of

	Breakfast		Lunch		Dinner		Night
	before	after	before	after	before	after	before
MONDAY							

Notes:

	before	after	before	after	before	after	before
TUESDAY							

Notes:

	before	after	before	after	before	after	before
WEDNESDAY							

Notes:

	before	after	before	after	before	after	before
THURSDAY							

Notes:

	before	after	before	after	before	after	before
FRIDAY							

Notes:

	before	after	before	after	before	after	before
SATURDAY							

Notes:

	before	after	before	after	before	after	before
SUNDAY							

Notes:

Week of

	Breakfast		Lunch		Dinner		Night
MONDAY	before	after	before	after	before	after	before
Notes:							
TUESDAY	before	after	before	after	before	after	before
Notes:							
WEDNESDAY	before	after	before	after	before	after	before
Notes:							
THURSDAY	before	after	before	after	before	after	before
Notes:							
FRIDAY	before	after	before	after	before	after	before
Notes:							
SATURDAY	before	after	before	after	before	after	before
Notes:							
SUNDAY	before	after	before	after	before	after	before
Notes:							

Week of

	Breakfast		Lunch		Dinner		Night
	before	after	before	after	before	after	before
MONDAY							

Notes:

	before	after	before	after	before	after	before
TUESDAY							

Notes:

	before	after	before	after	before	after	before
WEDNESDAY							

Notes:

	before	after	before	after	before	after	before
THURSDAY							

Notes:

	before	after	before	after	before	after	before
FRIDAY							

Notes:

	before	after	before	after	before	after	before
SATURDAY							

Notes:

	before	after	before	after	before	after	before
SUNDAY							

Notes:

Week of

	Breakfast		Lunch		Dinner		Night
	before	after	before	after	before	after	before
MONDAY							
Notes:							
TUESDAY	before	after	before	after	before	after	before
Notes:							
WEDNESDAY	before	after	before	after	before	after	before
Notes:							
THURSDAY	before	after	before	after	before	after	before
Notes:							
FRIDAY	before	after	before	after	before	after	before
Notes:							
SATURDAY	before	after	before	after	before	after	before
Notes:							
SUNDAY	before	after	before	after	before	after	before
Notes:							

Week of

	Breakfast		Lunch		Dinner		Night
	before	after	before	after	before	after	before
MONDAY							

Notes:

	before	after	before	after	before	after	before
TUESDAY							

Notes:

	before	after	before	after	before	after	before
WEDNESDAY							

Notes:

	before	after	before	after	before	after	before
THURSDAY							

Notes:

	before	after	before	after	before	after	before
FRIDAY							

Notes:

	before	after	before	after	before	after	before
SATURDAY							

Notes:

	before	after	before	after	before	after	before
SUNDAY							

Notes:

Week of

	Breakfast		Lunch		Dinner		Night
	before	after	before	after	before	after	before
MONDAY							

Notes:

	before	after	before	after	before	after	before
TUESDAY							

Notes:

	before	after	before	after	before	after	before
WEDNESDAY							

Notes:

	before	after	before	after	before	after	before
THURSDAY							

Notes:

	before	after	before	after	before	after	before
FRIDAY							

Notes:

	before	after	before	after	before	after	before
SATURDAY							

Notes:

	before	after	before	after	before	after	before
SUNDAY							

Notes:

Week of

	Breakfast		Lunch		Dinner		Night
	before	after	before	after	before	after	before
MONDAY							

Notes:

	before	after	before	after	before	after	before
TUESDAY							

Notes:

	before	after	before	after	before	after	before
WEDNESDAY							

Notes:

	before	after	before	after	before	after	before
THURSDAY							

Notes:

	before	after	before	after	before	after	before
FRIDAY							

Notes:

	before	after	before	after	before	after	before
SATURDAY							

Notes:

	before	after	before	after	before	after	before
SUNDAY							

Notes:

Week of

	Breakfast		Lunch		Dinner		Night
	before	after	before	after	before	after	before
MONDAY							

Notes:

	before	after	before	after	before	after	before
TUESDAY							

Notes:

	before	after	before	after	before	after	before
WEDNESDAY							

Notes:

	before	after	before	after	before	after	before
THURSDAY							

Notes:

	before	after	before	after	before	after	before
FRIDAY							

Notes:

	before	after	before	after	before	after	before
SATURDAY							

Notes:

	before	after	before	after	before	after	before
SUNDAY							

Notes:

Week of

	Breakfast		Lunch		Dinner		Night
	before	after	before	after	before	after	before
MONDAY							

Notes:

	before	after	before	after	before	after	before
TUESDAY							

Notes:

	before	after	before	after	before	after	before
WEDNESDAY							

Notes:

	before	after	before	after	before	after	before
THURSDAY							

Notes:

	before	after	before	after	before	after	before
FRIDAY							

Notes:

	before	after	before	after	before	after	before
SATURDAY							

Notes:

	before	after	before	after	before	after	before
SUNDAY							

Notes:

Week of

	Breakfast		Lunch		Dinner		Night
	before	after	before	after	before	after	before
MONDAY							

Notes:

	before	after	before	after	before	after	before
TUESDAY							

Notes:

	before	after	before	after	before	after	before
WEDNESDAY							

Notes:

	before	after	before	after	before	after	before
THURSDAY							

Notes:

	before	after	before	after	before	after	before
FRIDAY							

Notes:

	before	after	before	after	before	after	before
SATURDAY							

Notes:

	before	after	before	after	before	after	before
SUNDAY							

Notes:

Week of

	Breakfast		Lunch		Dinner		Night
	before	after	before	after	before	after	before
MONDAY							

Notes:

	before	after	before	after	before	after	before
TUESDAY							

Notes:

	before	after	before	after	before	after	before
WEDNESDAY							

Notes:

	before	after	before	after	before	after	before
THURSDAY							

Notes:

	before	after	before	after	before	after	before
FRIDAY							

Notes:

	before	after	before	after	before	after	before
SATURDAY							

Notes:

	before	after	before	after	before	after	before
SUNDAY							

Notes:

Week of

	Breakfast		Lunch		Dinner		Night
	before	after	before	after	before	after	before
MONDAY							

Notes:

	before	after	before	after	before	after	before
TUESDAY							

Notes:

	before	after	before	after	before	after	before
WEDNESDAY							

Notes:

	before	after	before	after	before	after	before
THURSDAY							

Notes:

	before	after	before	after	before	after	before
FRIDAY							

Notes:

	before	after	before	after	before	after	before
SATURDAY							

Notes:

	before	after	before	after	before	after	before
SUNDAY							

Notes:

Week of

	Breakfast		Lunch		Dinner		Night
	before	after	before	after	before	after	before
MONDAY							

Notes:

	before	after	before	after	before	after	before
TUESDAY							

Notes:

	before	after	before	after	before	after	before
WEDNESDAY							

Notes:

	before	after	before	after	before	after	before
THURSDAY							

Notes:

	before	after	before	after	before	after	before
FRIDAY							

Notes:

	before	after	before	after	before	after	before
SATURDAY							

Notes:

	before	after	before	after	before	after	before
SUNDAY							

Notes:

Week of

	Breakfast		Lunch		Dinner		Night
	before	after	before	after	before	after	before
MONDAY							

Notes:

	before	after	before	after	before	after	before
TUESDAY							

Notes:

	before	after	before	after	before	after	before
WEDNESDAY							

Notes:

	before	after	before	after	before	after	before
THURSDAY							

Notes:

	before	after	before	after	before	after	before
FRIDAY							

Notes:

	before	after	before	after	before	after	before
SATURDAY							

Notes:

	before	after	before	after	before	after	before
SUNDAY							

Notes:

Week of

	Breakfast		Lunch		Dinner		Night
	before	after	before	after	before	after	before
MONDAY							

Notes:

	before	after	before	after	before	after	before
TUESDAY							

Notes:

	before	after	before	after	before	after	before
WEDNESDAY							

Notes:

	before	after	before	after	before	after	before
THURSDAY							

Notes:

	before	after	before	after	before	after	before
FRIDAY							

Notes:

	before	after	before	after	before	after	before
SATURDAY							

Notes:

	before	after	before	after	before	after	before
SUNDAY							

Notes:

Week of

	Breakfast		Lunch		Dinner		Night
	before	after	before	after	before	after	before
MONDAY							

Notes:

	before	after	before	after	before	after	before
TUESDAY							

Notes:

	before	after	before	after	before	after	before
WEDNESDAY							

Notes:

	before	after	before	after	before	after	before
THURSDAY							

Notes:

	before	after	before	after	before	after	before
FRIDAY							

Notes:

	before	after	before	after	before	after	before
SATURDAY							

Notes:

	before	after	before	after	before	after	before
SUNDAY							

Notes:

Week of

	Breakfast		Lunch		Dinner		Night
	before	after	before	after	before	after	before
MONDAY							

Notes:

	before	after	before	after	before	after	before
TUESDAY							

Notes:

	before	after	before	after	before	after	before
WEDNESDAY							

Notes:

	before	after	before	after	before	after	before
THURSDAY							

Notes:

	before	after	before	after	before	after	before
FRIDAY							

Notes:

	before	after	before	after	before	after	before
SATURDAY							

Notes:

	before	after	before	after	before	after	before
SUNDAY							

Notes:

Week of

	Breakfast		Lunch		Dinner		Night
	before	after	before	after	before	after	before
MONDAY							

Notes:

	before	after	before	after	before	after	before
TUESDAY							

Notes:

	before	after	before	after	before	after	before
WEDNESDAY							

Notes:

	before	after	before	after	before	after	before
THURSDAY							

Notes:

	before	after	before	after	before	after	before
FRIDAY							

Notes:

	before	after	before	after	before	after	before
SATURDAY							

Notes:

	before	after	before	after	before	after	before
SUNDAY							

Notes:

Week of

	Breakfast		Lunch		Dinner		Night
	before	after	before	after	before	after	before
MONDAY							

Notes:

	before	after	before	after	before	after	before
TUESDAY							

Notes:

	before	after	before	after	before	after	before
WEDNESDAY							

Notes:

	before	after	before	after	before	after	before
THURSDAY							

Notes:

	before	after	before	after	before	after	before
FRIDAY							

Notes:

	before	after	before	after	before	after	before
SATURDAY							

Notes:

	before	after	before	after	before	after	before
SUNDAY							

Notes:

Week of

	Breakfast		Lunch		Dinner		Night
	before	after	before	after	before	after	before
MONDAY							

Notes:

	before	after	before	after	before	after	before
TUESDAY							

Notes:

	before	after	before	after	before	after	before
WEDNESDAY							

Notes:

	before	after	before	after	before	after	before
THURSDAY							

Notes:

	before	after	before	after	before	after	before
FRIDAY							

Notes:

	before	after	before	after	before	after	before
SATURDAY							

Notes:

	before	after	before	after	before	after	before
SUNDAY							

Notes:

Week of

	Breakfast		Lunch		Dinner		Night
	before	after	before	after	before	after	before
MONDAY							

Notes:

	before	after	before	after	before	after	before
TUESDAY							

Notes:

	before	after	before	after	before	after	before
WEDNESDAY							

Notes:

	before	after	before	after	before	after	before
THURSDAY							

Notes:

	before	after	before	after	before	after	before
FRIDAY							

Notes:

	before	after	before	after	before	after	before
SATURDAY							

Notes:

	before	after	before	after	before	after	before
SUNDAY							

Notes:

Week of

	Breakfast		Lunch		Dinner		Night
	before	after	before	after	before	after	before
MONDAY							

Notes:

	before	after	before	after	before	after	before
TUESDAY							

Notes:

	before	after	before	after	before	after	before
WEDNESDAY							

Notes:

	before	after	before	after	before	after	before
THURSDAY							

Notes:

	before	after	before	after	before	after	before
FRIDAY							

Notes:

	before	after	before	after	before	after	before
SATURDAY							

Notes:

	before	after	before	after	before	after	before
SUNDAY							

Notes:

Week of

	Breakfast		Lunch		Dinner		Night
	before	after	before	after	before	after	before
MONDAY							

Notes:

	before	after	before	after	before	after	before
TUESDAY							

Notes:

	before	after	before	after	before	after	before
WEDNESDAY							

Notes:

	before	after	before	after	before	after	before
THURSDAY							

Notes:

	before	after	before	after	before	after	before
FRIDAY							

Notes:

	before	after	before	after	before	after	before
SATURDAY							

Notes:

	before	after	before	after	before	after	before
SUNDAY							

Notes:

Week of

	Breakfast		Lunch		Dinner		Night
MONDAY	before	after	before	after	before	after	before

Notes:

	Breakfast		Lunch		Dinner		Night
TUESDAY	before	after	before	after	before	after	before

Notes:

	Breakfast		Lunch		Dinner		Night
WEDNESDAY	before	after	before	after	before	after	before

Notes:

	Breakfast		Lunch		Dinner		Night
THURSDAY	before	after	before	after	before	after	before

Notes:

	Breakfast		Lunch		Dinner		Night
FRIDAY	before	after	before	after	before	after	before

Notes:

	Breakfast		Lunch		Dinner		Night
SATURDAY	before	after	before	after	before	after	before

Notes:

	Breakfast		Lunch		Dinner		Night
SUNDAY	before	after	before	after	before	after	before

Notes:

Week of

	Breakfast		Lunch		Dinner		Night
	before	after	before	after	before	after	before
MONDAY							

Notes:

	before	after	before	after	before	after	before
TUESDAY							

Notes:

	before	after	before	after	before	after	before
WEDNESDAY							

Notes:

	before	after	before	after	before	after	before
THURSDAY							

Notes:

	before	after	before	after	before	after	before
FRIDAY							

Notes:

	before	after	before	after	before	after	before
SATURDAY							

Notes:

	before	after	before	after	before	after	before
SUNDAY							

Notes:

Week of

	Breakfast		Lunch		Dinner		Night
	before	after	before	after	before	after	before
MONDAY							

Notes:

	before	after	before	after	before	after	before
TUESDAY							

Notes:

	before	after	before	after	before	after	before
WEDNESDAY							

Notes:

	before	after	before	after	before	after	before
THURSDAY							

Notes:

	before	after	before	after	before	after	before
FRIDAY							

Notes:

	before	after	before	after	before	after	before
SATURDAY							

Notes:

	before	after	before	after	before	after	before
SUNDAY							

Notes:

Week of

	Breakfast		Lunch		Dinner		Night
	before	after	before	after	before	after	before
MONDAY							

Notes:

	before	after	before	after	before	after	before
TUESDAY							

Notes:

	before	after	before	after	before	after	before
WEDNESDAY							

Notes:

	before	after	before	after	before	after	before
THURSDAY							

Notes:

	before	after	before	after	before	after	before
FRIDAY							

Notes:

	before	after	before	after	before	after	before
SATURDAY							

Notes:

	before	after	before	after	before	after	before
SUNDAY							

Notes:

Week of

	Breakfast		Lunch		Dinner		Night
	before	after	before	after	before	after	before
MONDAY							

Notes:

	before	after	before	after	before	after	before
TUESDAY							

Notes:

	before	after	before	after	before	after	before
WEDNESDAY							

Notes:

	before	after	before	after	before	after	before
THURSDAY							

Notes:

	before	after	before	after	before	after	before
FRIDAY							

Notes:

	before	after	before	after	before	after	before
SATURDAY							

Notes:

	before	after	before	after	before	after	before
SUNDAY							

Notes:

Week of

	Breakfast		Lunch		Dinner		Night
	before	after	before	after	before	after	before
MONDAY							

Notes:

	before	after	before	after	before	after	before
TUESDAY							

Notes:

	before	after	before	after	before	after	before
WEDNESDAY							

Notes:

	before	after	before	after	before	after	before
THURSDAY							

Notes:

	before	after	before	after	before	after	before
FRIDAY							

Notes:

	before	after	before	after	before	after	before
SATURDAY							

Notes:

	before	after	before	after	before	after	before
SUNDAY							

Notes:

Week of

	Breakfast		Lunch		Dinner		Night
	before	after	before	after	before	after	before
MONDAY							

Notes:

	before	after	before	after	before	after	before
TUESDAY							

Notes:

	before	after	before	after	before	after	before
WEDNESDAY							

Notes:

	before	after	before	after	before	after	before
THURSDAY							

Notes:

	before	after	before	after	before	after	before
FRIDAY							

Notes:

	before	after	before	after	before	after	before
SATURDAY							

Notes:

	before	after	before	after	before	after	before
SUNDAY							

Notes:

Week of

	Breakfast		Lunch		Dinner		Night
	before	after	before	after	before	after	before
MONDAY							

Notes:

	before	after	before	after	before	after	before
TUESDAY							

Notes:

	before	after	before	after	before	after	before
WEDNESDAY							

Notes:

	before	after	before	after	before	after	before
THURSDAY							

Notes:

	before	after	before	after	before	after	before
FRIDAY							

Notes:

	before	after	before	after	before	after	before
SATURDAY							

Notes:

	before	after	before	after	before	after	before
SUNDAY							

Notes:

Week of

	Breakfast		Lunch		Dinner		Night
	before	after	before	after	before	after	before
MONDAY							

Notes:

	before	after	before	after	before	after	before
TUESDAY							

Notes:

	before	after	before	after	before	after	before
WEDNESDAY							

Notes:

	before	after	before	after	before	after	before
THURSDAY							

Notes:

	before	after	before	after	before	after	before
FRIDAY							

Notes:

	before	after	before	after	before	after	before
SATURDAY							

Notes:

	before	after	before	after	before	after	before
SUNDAY							

Notes:

Week of

	Breakfast		Lunch		Dinner		Night
	before	after	before	after	before	after	before
MONDAY							

Notes:

	before	after	before	after	before	after	before
TUESDAY							

Notes:

	before	after	before	after	before	after	before
WEDNESDAY							

Notes:

	before	after	before	after	before	after	before
THURSDAY							

Notes:

	before	after	before	after	before	after	before
FRIDAY							

Notes:

	before	after	before	after	before	after	before
SATURDAY							

Notes:

	before	after	before	after	before	after	before
SUNDAY							

Notes:

Week of

	Breakfast		Lunch		Dinner		Night
	before	after	before	after	before	after	before
MONDAY							

Notes:

	before	after	before	after	before	after	before
TUESDAY							

Notes:

	before	after	before	after	before	after	before
WEDNESDAY							

Notes:

	before	after	before	after	before	after	before
THURSDAY							

Notes:

	before	after	before	after	before	after	before
FRIDAY							

Notes:

	before	after	before	after	before	after	before
SATURDAY							

Notes:

	before	after	before	after	before	after	before
SUNDAY							

Notes:

Week of

	Breakfast		Lunch		Dinner		Night
	before	after	before	after	before	after	before
MONDAY							

Notes:

	before	after	before	after	before	after	before
TUESDAY							

Notes:

	before	after	before	after	before	after	before
WEDNESDAY							

Notes:

	before	after	before	after	before	after	before
THURSDAY							

Notes:

	before	after	before	after	before	after	before
FRIDAY							

Notes:

	before	after	before	after	before	after	before
SATURDAY							

Notes:

	before	after	before	after	before	after	before
SUNDAY							

Notes:

Week of

	Breakfast		Lunch		Dinner		Night
	before	after	before	after	before	after	before
MONDAY							

Notes:

	before	after	before	after	before	after	before
TUESDAY							

Notes:

	before	after	before	after	before	after	before
WEDNESDAY							

Notes:

	before	after	before	after	before	after	before
THURSDAY							

Notes:

	before	after	before	after	before	after	before
FRIDAY							

Notes:

	before	after	before	after	before	after	before
SATURDAY							

Notes:

	before	after	before	after	before	after	before
SUNDAY							

Notes:

Week of

	Breakfast		Lunch		Dinner		Night
	before	after	before	after	before	after	before
MONDAY							

Notes:

	before	after	before	after	before	after	before
TUESDAY							

Notes:

	before	after	before	after	before	after	before
WEDNESDAY							

Notes:

	before	after	before	after	before	after	before
THURSDAY							

Notes:

	before	after	before	after	before	after	before
FRIDAY							

Notes:

	before	after	before	after	before	after	before
SATURDAY							

Notes:

	before	after	before	after	before	after	before
SUNDAY							

Notes:

Week of

	Breakfast		Lunch		Dinner		Night
	before	after	before	after	before	after	before
MONDAY							
Notes:							
TUESDAY	before	after	before	after	before	after	before
Notes:							
WEDNESDAY	before	after	before	after	before	after	before
Notes:							
THURSDAY	before	after	before	after	before	after	before
Notes:							
FRIDAY	before	after	before	after	before	after	before
Notes:							
SATURDAY	before	after	before	after	before	after	before
Notes:							
SUNDAY	before	after	before	after	before	after	before
Notes:							

Week of

	Breakfast		Lunch		Dinner		Night
	before	after	before	after	before	after	before
MONDAY							

Notes:

	before	after	before	after	before	after	before
TUESDAY							

Notes:

	before	after	before	after	before	after	before
WEDNESDAY							

Notes:

	before	after	before	after	before	after	before
THURSDAY							

Notes:

	before	after	before	after	before	after	before
FRIDAY							

Notes:

	before	after	before	after	before	after	before
SATURDAY							

Notes:

	before	after	before	after	before	after	before
SUNDAY							

Notes:

Week of

	Breakfast		Lunch		Dinner		Night
	before	after	before	after	before	after	before
MONDAY							

Notes:

	before	after	before	after	before	after	before
TUESDAY							

Notes:

	before	after	before	after	before	after	before
WEDNESDAY							

Notes:

	before	after	before	after	before	after	before
THURSDAY							

Notes:

	before	after	before	after	before	after	before
FRIDAY							

Notes:

	before	after	before	after	before	after	before
SATURDAY							

Notes:

	before	after	before	after	before	after	before
SUNDAY							

Notes:

Week of

	Breakfast		Lunch		Dinner		Night
	before	after	before	after	before	after	before
MONDAY							

Notes:

	before	after	before	after	before	after	before
TUESDAY							

Notes:

	before	after	before	after	before	after	before
WEDNESDAY							

Notes:

	before	after	before	after	before	after	before
THURSDAY							

Notes:

	before	after	before	after	before	after	before
FRIDAY							

Notes:

	before	after	before	after	before	after	before
SATURDAY							

Notes:

	before	after	before	after	before	after	before
SUNDAY							

Notes:

Week of

	Breakfast		Lunch		Dinner		Night
	before	after	before	after	before	after	before
MONDAY							

Notes:

	before	after	before	after	before	after	before
TUESDAY							

Notes:

	before	after	before	after	before	after	before
WEDNESDAY							

Notes:

	before	after	before	after	before	after	before
THURSDAY							

Notes:

	before	after	before	after	before	after	before
FRIDAY							

Notes:

	before	after	before	after	before	after	before
SATURDAY							

Notes:

	before	after	before	after	before	after	before
SUNDAY							

Notes:

Week of

	Breakfast		Lunch		Dinner		Night
	before	after	before	after	before	after	before
MONDAY							

Notes:

	before	after	before	after	before	after	before
TUESDAY							

Notes:

	before	after	before	after	before	after	before
WEDNESDAY							

Notes:

	before	after	before	after	before	after	before
THURSDAY							

Notes:

	before	after	before	after	before	after	before
FRIDAY							

Notes:

	before	after	before	after	before	after	before
SATURDAY							

Notes:

	before	after	before	after	before	after	before
SUNDAY							

Notes:

Week of

	Breakfast		Lunch		Dinner		Night
	before	after	before	after	before	after	before
MONDAY							

Notes:

	before	after	before	after	before	after	before
TUESDAY							

Notes:

	before	after	before	after	before	after	before
WEDNESDAY							

Notes:

	before	after	before	after	before	after	before
THURSDAY							

Notes:

	before	after	before	after	before	after	before
FRIDAY							

Notes:

	before	after	before	after	before	after	before
SATURDAY							

Notes:

	before	after	before	after	before	after	before
SUNDAY							

Notes:

Week of

	Breakfast		Lunch		Dinner		Night
	before	after	before	after	before	after	before
MONDAY							

Notes:

	before	after	before	after	before	after	before
TUESDAY							

Notes:

	before	after	before	after	before	after	before
WEDNESDAY							

Notes:

	before	after	before	after	before	after	before
THURSDAY							

Notes:

	before	after	before	after	before	after	before
FRIDAY							

Notes:

	before	after	before	after	before	after	before
SATURDAY							

Notes:

	before	after	before	after	before	after	before
SUNDAY							

Notes:

Week of

	Breakfast		Lunch		Dinner		Night
	before	after	before	after	before	after	before
MONDAY							

Notes:

	before	after	before	after	before	after	before
TUESDAY							

Notes:

	before	after	before	after	before	after	before
WEDNESDAY							

Notes:

	before	after	before	after	before	after	before
THURSDAY							

Notes:

	before	after	before	after	before	after	before
FRIDAY							

Notes:

	before	after	before	after	before	after	before
SATURDAY							

Notes:

	before	after	before	after	before	after	before
SUNDAY							

Notes:

Week of

	Breakfast		Lunch		Dinner		Night
	before	after	before	after	before	after	before
MONDAY							

Notes:

	before	after	before	after	before	after	before
TUESDAY							

Notes:

	before	after	before	after	before	after	before
WEDNESDAY							

Notes:

	before	after	before	after	before	after	before
THURSDAY							

Notes:

	before	after	before	after	before	after	before
FRIDAY							

Notes:

	before	after	before	after	before	after	before
SATURDAY							

Notes:

	before	after	before	after	before	after	before
SUNDAY							

Notes:

Week of

	Breakfast		Lunch		Dinner		Night
MONDAY	before	after	before	after	before	after	before
Notes:							
TUESDAY	before	after	before	after	before	after	before
Notes:							
WEDNESDAY	before	after	before	after	before	after	before
Notes:							
THURSDAY	before	after	before	after	before	after	before
Notes:							
FRIDAY	before	after	before	after	before	after	before
Notes:							
SATURDAY	before	after	before	after	before	after	before
Notes:							
SUNDAY	before	after	before	after	before	after	before
Notes:							

Week of

	Breakfast		Lunch		Dinner		Night
	before	after	before	after	before	after	before
MONDAY							

Notes:

	before	after	before	after	before	after	before
TUESDAY							

Notes:

	before	after	before	after	before	after	before
WEDNESDAY							

Notes:

	before	after	before	after	before	after	before
THURSDAY							

Notes:

	before	after	before	after	before	after	before
FRIDAY							

Notes:

	before	after	before	after	before	after	before
SATURDAY							

Notes:

	before	after	before	after	before	after	before
SUNDAY							

Notes:

Week of

	Breakfast		Lunch		Dinner		Night
	before	after	before	after	before	after	before
MONDAY							

Notes:

	before	after	before	after	before	after	before
TUESDAY							

Notes:

	before	after	before	after	before	after	before
WEDNESDAY							

Notes:

	before	after	before	after	before	after	before
THURSDAY							

Notes:

	before	after	before	after	before	after	before
FRIDAY							

Notes:

	before	after	before	after	before	after	before
SATURDAY							

Notes:

	before	after	before	after	before	after	before
SUNDAY							

Notes:

Week of

	Breakfast		Lunch		Dinner		Night
	before	after	before	after	before	after	before
MONDAY							

Notes:

	before	after	before	after	before	after	before
TUESDAY							

Notes:

	before	after	before	after	before	after	before
WEDNESDAY							

Notes:

	before	after	before	after	before	after	before
THURSDAY							

Notes:

	before	after	before	after	before	after	before
FRIDAY							

Notes:

	before	after	before	after	before	after	before
SATURDAY							

Notes:

	before	after	before	after	before	after	before
SUNDAY							

Notes:

Week of

	Breakfast		Lunch		Dinner		Night
	before	after	before	after	before	after	before
MONDAY							

Notes:

	before	after	before	after	before	after	before
TUESDAY							

Notes:

	before	after	before	after	before	after	before
WEDNESDAY							

Notes:

	before	after	before	after	before	after	before
THURSDAY							

Notes:

	before	after	before	after	before	after	before
FRIDAY							

Notes:

	before	after	before	after	before	after	before
SATURDAY							

Notes:

	before	after	before	after	before	after	before
SUNDAY							

Notes:

Week of

	Breakfast		Lunch		Dinner		Night
	before	after	before	after	before	after	before
MONDAY							

Notes:

	before	after	before	after	before	after	before
TUESDAY							

Notes:

	before	after	before	after	before	after	before
WEDNESDAY							

Notes:

	before	after	before	after	before	after	before
THURSDAY							

Notes:

	before	after	before	after	before	after	before
FRIDAY							

Notes:

	before	after	before	after	before	after	before
SATURDAY							

Notes:

	before	after	before	after	before	after	before
SUNDAY							

Notes:

Week of

	Breakfast		Lunch		Dinner		Night
	before	after	before	after	before	after	before
MONDAY							

Notes:

	before	after	before	after	before	after	before
TUESDAY							

Notes:

	before	after	before	after	before	after	before
WEDNESDAY							

Notes:

	before	after	before	after	before	after	before
THURSDAY							

Notes:

	before	after	before	after	before	after	before
FRIDAY							

Notes:

	before	after	before	after	before	after	before
SATURDAY							

Notes:

	before	after	before	after	before	after	before
SUNDAY							

Notes:

Week of

	Breakfast		Lunch		Dinner		Night
	before	after	before	after	before	after	before
MONDAY							

Notes:

	before	after	before	after	before	after	before
TUESDAY							

Notes:

	before	after	before	after	before	after	before
WEDNESDAY							

Notes:

	before	after	before	after	before	after	before
THURSDAY							

Notes:

	before	after	before	after	before	after	before
FRIDAY							

Notes:

	before	after	before	after	before	after	before
SATURDAY							

Notes:

	before	after	before	after	before	after	before
SUNDAY							

Notes:

Week of

	Breakfast		Lunch		Dinner		Night
	before	after	before	after	before	after	before
MONDAY							

Notes:

	before	after	before	after	before	after	before
TUESDAY							

Notes:

	before	after	before	after	before	after	before
WEDNESDAY							

Notes:

	before	after	before	after	before	after	before
THURSDAY							

Notes:

	before	after	before	after	before	after	before
FRIDAY							

Notes:

	before	after	before	after	before	after	before
SATURDAY							

Notes:

	before	after	before	after	before	after	before
SUNDAY							

Notes:

Week of

	Breakfast		Lunch		Dinner		Night
	before	after	before	after	before	after	before
MONDAY							

Notes:

	before	after	before	after	before	after	before
TUESDAY							

Notes:

	before	after	before	after	before	after	before
WEDNESDAY							

Notes:

	before	after	before	after	before	after	before
THURSDAY							

Notes:

	before	after	before	after	before	after	before
FRIDAY							

Notes:

	before	after	before	after	before	after	before
SATURDAY							

Notes:

	before	after	before	after	before	after	before
SUNDAY							

Notes:

Week of

	Breakfast		Lunch		Dinner		Night
	before	after	before	after	before	after	before
MONDAY							

Notes:

	before	after	before	after	before	after	before
TUESDAY							

Notes:

	before	after	before	after	before	after	before
WEDNESDAY							

Notes:

	before	after	before	after	before	after	before
THURSDAY							

Notes:

	before	after	before	after	before	after	before
FRIDAY							

Notes:

	before	after	before	after	before	after	before
SATURDAY							

Notes:

	before	after	before	after	before	after	before
SUNDAY							

Notes:

Week of

	Breakfast		Lunch		Dinner		Night
	before	after	before	after	before	after	before
MONDAY							

Notes:

	before	after	before	after	before	after	before
TUESDAY							

Notes:

	before	after	before	after	before	after	before
WEDNESDAY							

Notes:

	before	after	before	after	before	after	before
THURSDAY							

Notes:

	before	after	before	after	before	after	before
FRIDAY							

Notes:

	before	after	before	after	before	after	before
SATURDAY							

Notes:

	before	after	before	after	before	after	before
SUNDAY							

Notes:

Week of

	Breakfast		Lunch		Dinner		Night
	before	after	before	after	before	after	before
MONDAY							

Notes:

	before	after	before	after	before	after	before
TUESDAY							

Notes:

	before	after	before	after	before	after	before
WEDNESDAY							

Notes:

	before	after	before	after	before	after	before
THURSDAY							

Notes:

	before	after	before	after	before	after	before
FRIDAY							

Notes:

	before	after	before	after	before	after	before
SATURDAY							

Notes:

	before	after	before	after	before	after	before
SUNDAY							

Notes:

Week of

	Breakfast		Lunch		Dinner		Night
	before	after	before	after	before	after	before
MONDAY							

Notes:

	before	after	before	after	before	after	before
TUESDAY							

Notes:

	before	after	before	after	before	after	before
WEDNESDAY							

Notes:

	before	after	before	after	before	after	before
THURSDAY							

Notes:

	before	after	before	after	before	after	before
FRIDAY							

Notes:

	before	after	before	after	before	after	before
SATURDAY							

Notes:

	before	after	before	after	before	after	before
SUNDAY							

Notes:

Week of

	Breakfast		Lunch		Dinner		Night
	before	after	before	after	before	after	before
MONDAY							

Notes:

	before	after	before	after	before	after	before
TUESDAY							

Notes:

	before	after	before	after	before	after	before
WEDNESDAY							

Notes:

	before	after	before	after	before	after	before
THURSDAY							

Notes:

	before	after	before	after	before	after	before
FRIDAY							

Notes:

	before	after	before	after	before	after	before
SATURDAY							

Notes:

	before	after	before	after	before	after	before
SUNDAY							

Notes:

Week of

	Breakfast		Lunch		Dinner		Night
	before	after	before	after	before	after	before
MONDAY							

Notes:

	before	after	before	after	before	after	before
TUESDAY							

Notes:

	before	after	before	after	before	after	before
WEDNESDAY							

Notes:

	before	after	before	after	before	after	before
THURSDAY							

Notes:

	before	after	before	after	before	after	before
FRIDAY							

Notes:

	before	after	before	after	before	after	before
SATURDAY							

Notes:

	before	after	before	after	before	after	before
SUNDAY							

Notes:

Week of

	Breakfast		Lunch		Dinner		Night
	before	after	before	after	before	after	before
MONDAY							
Notes:							
TUESDAY	before	after	before	after	before	after	before
Notes:							
WEDNESDAY	before	after	before	after	before	after	before
Notes:							
THURSDAY	before	after	before	after	before	after	before
Notes:							
FRIDAY	before	after	before	after	before	after	before
Notes:							
SATURDAY	before	after	before	after	before	after	before
Notes:							
SUNDAY	before	after	before	after	before	after	before
Notes:							

Week of

	Breakfast		Lunch		Dinner		Night
	before	after	before	after	before	after	before
MONDAY							

Notes:

	before	after	before	after	before	after	before
TUESDAY							

Notes:

	before	after	before	after	before	after	before
WEDNESDAY							

Notes:

	before	after	before	after	before	after	before
THURSDAY							

Notes:

	before	after	before	after	before	after	before
FRIDAY							

Notes:

	before	after	before	after	before	after	before
SATURDAY							

Notes:

	before	after	before	after	before	after	before
SUNDAY							

Notes:

Week of

	Breakfast		Lunch		Dinner		Night
	before	after	before	after	before	after	before
MONDAY							
Notes:							
TUESDAY	before	after	before	after	before	after	before
Notes:							
WEDNESDAY	before	after	before	after	before	after	before
Notes:							
THURSDAY	before	after	before	after	before	after	before
Notes:							
FRIDAY	before	after	before	after	before	after	before
Notes:							
SATURDAY	before	after	before	after	before	after	before
Notes:							
SUNDAY	before	after	before	after	before	after	before
Notes:							

Week of

	Breakfast		Lunch		Dinner		Night
	before	after	before	after	before	after	before
MONDAY							

Notes:

	before	after	before	after	before	after	before
TUESDAY							

Notes:

	before	after	before	after	before	after	before
WEDNESDAY							

Notes:

	before	after	before	after	before	after	before
THURSDAY							

Notes:

	before	after	before	after	before	after	before
FRIDAY							

Notes:

	before	after	before	after	before	after	before
SATURDAY							

Notes:

	before	after	before	after	before	after	before
SUNDAY							

Notes:

Printed in Great Britain
by Amazon